I0838039

Set Your House in Order

For You Shall Live!

A Story of Surviving
Terminal Cancer

James A. "Hoss" Boyd, LtCol, USAF
(Retired)

2 Kings 20:1-5
NKJV

In those days Hezekiah was sick and near death. And Isaiah the prophet, the son of Amoz, went to him and said to him, "Thus says the Lord: 'Set your house in order, for you shall die, and not live.' "

Then he turned his face to the wall, and prayed unto the Lord, saying, I beseech thee, O Lord, remember now how I have walked before thee in truth and with a perfect heart, and have done that which is good in thy sight. And Hezekiah wept sore.

And it came to pass, before Isaiah was gone out into the middle court, that the word of the Lord came to him, saying, "Turn again, and tell Hezekiah the captain of my people, "Thus saith the Lord, the God of David thy father, I have heard thy prayer, I have seen thy tears: behold, I will heal thee".

LEGAL

Set Your House In Order For You Shall Live!
Copyright © 2024 James A. "Hoss" Boyd, LtCol, USAF
(Retired). All rights retained. Reproduction of this
material is prohibited in any form except by the
express permission of the author.

This book is intended to inspire. It is shared with the
understanding that neither the author nor the
publisher is engaged in rendering legal, financial,
medical, or other professional advice. The author
and the publisher specifically disclaim any liability
that is incurred from the use or application of the
contents of this book.

Although a true story, certain events and
characters in the book have been changed or
omitted to protect the privacy of the individuals.

Authored and Published by James A. "Hoss" Boyd,
LtCol, USAF (Retired)

DEDICATION

Someone once said that no one on their death bed ever prayed for more time to spend at their career or hobby. In most cases, they regret not spending enough time with those they love. This is dedicated to my family, my wife Geneva, my daughter Missy, and my son James; and all those other families who have had to endure the hardships of a serious illness or pending death of a loved one and praying that they will be granted more time to spend with each other.

Acknowledgment
By
Dr. William T. Luffman
Senior Founding Pastor
Faith Outreach Church,
Clarksville, Tennessee

I believe that you are reading this book because the Holy Spirit is directing you to do so. Hopefully, you will never have to read it because you identify with its subject matter personally. But odds are, if not, one or more of your family members and/or close friends have.

After reading *"Set Your House in Order For You Shall Live – A Story of Surviving Cancer"*, I was struck by three amazing revelations:

First of all, the insidious malady of Cancer and how it can be so well hidden before it is discovered. By the time of discovery, it is often too late. It's effect on more than just the patient is also another piece of its insidiousness. In this book, Hoss gives the reader a very personal inside look at how cancer can be so interrupting and invasive in a person and families lives. He describes in great detail the "nature of the beast", and its unrelenting impact on the human body.

Secondly, Mr. Boyd gives those who are aware of military life, a vivid picture of how that translates into decision making and planning where the family is concerned.   For those of us who are civilian, like myself, we get a very clear understanding of the unusual stress and strain that military personnel and families endure.

And third, the incredible things that happen when medicine and faith are not divided or poised against each other, but are rather, blended together!   This "dynamic duo" becomes an unbeatable recipe for a miracle!

I believe this book is a God-send! May it inspire you and cause you to seek a deeper spiritual walk with God, so that when you are faced with a trial, you know how to mix your faith into the situation and come out victorious!

I highly recommend this book to everyone!

Sincerely,
Dr. William T. Luffman
Senior Founding Pastor
Faith Outreach Church,
Clarksville, Tennessee

Forward
By
Ray Still, Senior Pastor
Oakwood Baptist Church
New Braunfels, Texas

We learn so much from stories. Not only do we learn about individuals, but we also learn about ourselves. The problem that we have so often here in our society is that we do not stop and read or listen to those stories. But when we do, understanding, empathy and encouragement to live higher and better often comes. As what I think you will receive, if you invest the time to read Hoss' story. You will gain great understanding and you will be encouraged concerning God's faithfulness. After a reading of Hoss' work, there is only one verse that God reminds me of from the Apostle Paul concerning his thorn in the flesh. 2 Corinthians 12:9, Jesus tells him, "My grace is sufficient for you and my power is made perfect in weakness". You will see in Hoss' story, the sufficiency of God's grace and the power of God in a man's life. It has been my privilege over the past decades to be Hoss's and his family's Pastor. After reading his work, I found myself understanding and encouraged of what God has done in his life. Take the time to read and listen.

INTRODUCTION
By
James A. "Hoss" Boyd, LtCol, USAF (Retired)

As I write this, I am decades past my 38th birthday, and I am looking forward to many more productive years. But my story after my 38th birthday may never have been written. In 1988, Geneva, my young wife of 14 years of marriage, was told by my doctor to get our house in order. I can't imagine how hard those words had hit her, but the idea of being a young widow with two pre-teen children had to be traumatic. But as Mark Twain was famously quoted, "the report of my death has been grossly exaggerated." Although in truth, I shouldn't be here to share this story, God had other plans for me.

I was never told about my "terminal" condition until I had fully recovered. In fact, it wasn't until I wrote this Testimonial that I found out from Geneva how close to death I really was. It probably wouldn't have mattered if I had known, as I chose to believe that only God knows the time of our last moments on earth, and I knew that it wasn't my time---I had too much to live for. At the time, I was going through many seemingly insurmountable challenges. I was too focused on my problems to realize what my wife, daughter, and son were going through those problems as well. Everyone facing challenges --- whether they be financial, marital, or something as serious as cancer --- regardless of the hardship, one should never forget that their family is also suffering.

The road to recovery for me was far from easy, but of all the promises God makes, it is that He will give us strength to get through the tough times if we are willing to accept Him and believe. This is Geneva's, Missy's, James', and my story of a family surviving "terminal" cancer and our encouragement to others facing death from cancer or any other life-threatening condition; and the families of those affected---which at last accounting is eventually everyone.

Table of Contents

Part 1
The Clock Ticks Down

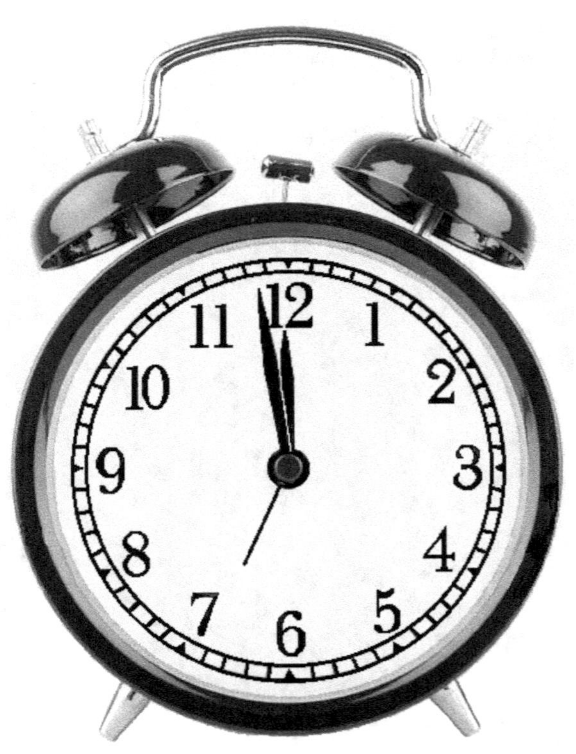

Part 1
The Clock Ticks Down

Imagine, if you will, a big clock (the old-fashioned analog kind with numbers 1 to 12, a big hand, and a little one). Assume that 12:00 noon is when cancer starts to grow inside of you. As your "cancer" clock ticks away, you don't notice anything at all at first. By the time the little hand is on the six, you may notice getting a little tired after doing routine activities, and possibly a few cuts or scrapes that seem to take a little longer to heal. You start to get concerned when the little hand is on 10:00 and you finally see a doctor for what you believe is the flu or some unusual pains you hadn't noticed before. The doctor accepts your diagnosis of a virus and sends you home to take aspirin and drink lots of fluids. At 11:00 PM you are having pains of greater intensity and possibly some unexplained bleeding. In my case, the pain and bleeding were attributed to an ulcer, since I was in a high stress situation and was too young to be the typical colon cancer patient.   The reality was much different. I was dying and was scheduled to do so when the clock struck midnight! You might say I was in that final countdown hour with two symbolic minutes left to live, when I was hospitalized under emergency conditions. I was just 38 years old, so how did it happen that an otherwise healthy young man in the prime of his life should be facing a certain death?

****

    Military life is stress at extreme levels for both the military members and their families. The hours can be very long and the demands on an individual so great that one is stretched to the absolute limit. As I neared the end of my second assignment while stationed in Alaska, I was faced with a career plagued with bad superiors, highly demanding jobs that were important but not promotable, and a military that was thinning the ranks. There I was with a young wife and two preschoolers who depended upon me for their livelihood and protection. I believed myself to be in great condition at the time; after all, I was benching over 300 pounds and running up to 6 miles at a stretch. But then there were those tell-tale signs: periods of being washed out physically, a declining bench press, sores that would appear for no apparent reason and take a long time to go away, and occasionally just being in a mental fog.

    One of the clever tricks the military used to keep people on active duty was their requirement that you had to forecast your voluntary separation 12 months ahead of time. However, most employers in the late 1970's were hiring a maximum of 30-60 days in advance of when they wanted the new hire to start work. With me being in Alaska and the jobs back in the lower 48, the logistics of a job search wasn't going to be practical. So, there I was with a young family and still saving for our first house; I just couldn't risk putting in my paperwork that far in advance without knowing I had a job to go to.

My solution was to stay on active duty and change career fields to one that was promotable. I volunteered for Titan II Missile duty, a job that was even more stressful, as well as potentially dangerous. The plan was a good one. We'd move to Little Rock, Arkansas; closer to home, family, and people I knew; put in my four years of missile crew duty; then transition from there to a civilian job. What I didn't consider was the huge reduction I would take in a paycheck if I separated and the number of years I would have invested in a career by the time the four-year missile tour was up. There was also the good possibility I would get promoted, and by all indications, I was in a highly promotable career field for a change.

****

For the first time in my military career, I had found my niche. I had always been fascinated with gadgets (I still am!!), and what a great treasure trove of gadgets a kid like me could find in a Titan II Missile Complex!!! I became an expert very quickly, plus I had led organizations with as many as 80 people. Being a Senior Captain, I was pushed rapidly upward through the various crew positions, eventually becoming an instructor and an evaluator. In a heartbeat, this all changed that fateful day in August of 1980. I was the commander of a special missile complex known as the Alternate Command Post (ACP). The site was one of two equipped with unique communications equipment so that in the event of a nuclear attack on the main base, my site could take over command and control of the other missile complexes. If my site was taken out, then the other unique site would be next in line. Although that alert tour started out like most others, the peace would be interrupted when a maintenance crew at another missile complex (Damascus, Arkansas, Complex 374-7), dropped a 5-inch socket tool. The tool fell over 100 feet before ricocheting into the Titan's fuel tank causing an uncontrollable rocket fuel leak followed several hours later by a catastrophic explosion. One airman was killed in the accident and several others injured. My crew and I were at a safe distance about an hour away, and able to monitor the situation to some extent through our special communications gear. This would be known as the most serious nuclear weapon related accident in our military history. One of the ironic aspects of that episode was the site I was assigned to that day was 373-7 (same site number but a different squadron). But even more ironic, that same maintenance crew started their day at my site first doing the same procedure with the same 5-inch socket tool. Another "Thank You

God" event that they didn't drop the socket tool at my site.

I would never trivialize the loss of life or the shortened lives of those who died young from breathing the toxic fumes. But the accident also had a devastating effect on almost everyone's careers---mostly in a negative way. Mine was no exception. To make sure we would all be a more responsible missile wing, all the senior leadership was summarily replaced and those of us who were in senior line positions like myself were replaced by the new commander's favorite people who he brought with him to Little Rock. It didn't help that literally everyone who had diligently worked their way up the operations ladder from the bottom rung of line crew was associated with the old leadership, and that included me in a significant way. So over a short period of time, it was out with the old and in with the new; not very good timing with a promotion board right around the corner. Added to the uncertainty of my upcoming promotion board in an "up-or-out" system, the stress levels multiplied because of increased hours of intensified remedial training, and added requirements at the missile sites.

****

Now let me take a step back. I have been a "Believer" all my life, although there were times when I was a stronger Christian than others. This was a time in my life when I was letting the affairs of the world take priority. I was taught to have faith that "all things are possible through Christ". I had the belief, but I was trying to do everything on my own without asking God for his infinite wisdom and anointing. There were many times when God opened the right doors for me but I was either too proud or too stupid to walk through them. A good rule of thumb, I learned, is that people who consistently make stupid decisions don't live as long as those who make good decisions. The way I was going, I was destined to literally have a very short life span. How much different it might have been had I just given it all up to God in the first place!

Things went from bad to worse when I chose what I thought would be a primo assignment in Albuquerque. That was the nail that sealed my coffin (so to speak). It was just like the old cowboy saying (paraphrased), "There's a lot they didn't tell me when I signed on with this outfit." After a frustrating two years at the new job in a city I wasn't familiar with, I decided to accept a fairly nice severance from the military. That would have been the perfect time to move back home and start fresh, but instead I made the next big mistake (in the missile world, they would call it a "Critical Error"). I dove headfirst into the local real estate industry with no training, no experience, and no business base---just before the big real estate crash of the early 1980's. Another major career decision without the benefit of God's anointing. It was shortly afterwards that severe abdominal pain and internal bleeding signaled a serious problem.

****

Adding to my worsening health condition, was a dwindling bank account, a new mortgage payment, the pressures of feeding and clothing my family, and no job or prospects of any. That's when I finally realized God was in control and He wanted my total attention. Sometimes He speaks through that still small voice, but other times, like in my case, He has to beat you down until you finally give it all up to Him.

Geneva was still working, but her paycheck was barely covering the bills. After an especially tight month, we only had $50 to our name. Christmas that year was especially depressing. Years later I found a "Letter to Santa" my daughter, Missy, had written back then. It read, "Dear Santa, Daddy and Mommie don't have money for presents this year, so if you could just bring them something, I would really 'preciate it." How often do we forget that hard times effect every member of the family---not just the parents.

Thank goodness I chose to stay connected to the military. Geneva had encouraged me to go into the Active Reserves---one of the times I really listened to someone. Weekend tours once a month didn't pay a lot but it did help out, and when the office learned I was available all the time, they found ways to keep me on short-term active duty gigs. On one particular day when we had zeroed out our bank account well before the next pay day, I remember praying a prayer of desperation with tears streaming down my face. At the time, I was headed to the Air Force Base to check on possible additional duty. I prayed that God would open up a door---any door---that would get us over that financial crisis. As I now live and breathe, I can testify that God does answer prayers. That was on a Friday, on Monday I was in Fort Worth, Texas, starting a temporary but high paying job for the organization. The colonel in charge of the department I was assigned to for my reserve duty just happened to need at that very time, a temporary replacement in a critical position, and he needed it filled immediately. That was the first of many answers to prayers. For once, I had listened to God's call and promptly volunteered for the job. It would mean only a few short months of separation, and during those months I could look for something more permanent. Then, I would be able to either move back with my family and start a new (and high paying) job with career possibilities or find something in Texas.

Instead of a year away in Ft. Worth, I was there only about six months before a permanent government job opened up back in Albuquerque. That meant I could be back with my family much sooner and we wouldn't have to sell our house at a huge loss. <u>God was answering my prayers when I gave it all up to Him.</u> Even the abdominal pains appeared to have faded away.

****

All seemed to be going great. I loved the new job in Albuquerque, and had a really great group of people to work with. In a short period of time, I was moved up in the organization where I found the duties both challenging and rewarding. Then God threw another mountain in front of me; the abdominal pains returned with a vengeance. This time, I would get sick to my stomach eating the blandest of foods---even tap water would make me nauseous. This would be followed with violent and frequent abdominal spasms that would double me over with pain. At the same time, it was becoming harder for me to be productive both at home and at work.

By Thanksgiving, the abdominal pains were coming every few minutes like labor pains. It was so bad that I totally passed on Thanksgiving Dinner and just laid on the couch bent over like a pretzel while everyone else enjoyed the turkey and all the "fixin's". I had been seeing a doctor for a couple of years who didn't think anything serious was going on, and it was evident he wasn't going to be much help. But instead of seeking the advice of other doctors, I just lingered on without the medical attention I desperately needed.

Shortly after the New Year, things became critical. Somehow, I made it through one of the worst nights of my life---I was totally blocked and my abdomen had doubled in size overnight. Geneva and I both knew something serious was going on when I started throwing up blood. But again, instead of realizing this was an emergency and we should be calling an ambulance, I convinced Geneva to just wait until I could see a doctor later that morning.

Despite the fact that I was literally dying, God was still watching out for me. The old doctor had dropped off of our medical plan and we had just changed doctors; that day was my first visit. The new doctor, Dr. Robert Foreman*, told my wife to get me to the emergency room immediately! I would bet the former doctor would have prescribed an antacid and sent me home where I would have surely died.

I can't say enough about how much we appreciate Dr. Robert Foreman of Albuquerque NM (now retired) who knew I needed immediate attention and worked behind the scenes during that crucial period to make sure I had the right team of doctors.

I was able to track down Dr. Foreman and let him know I was still around and how grateful I was for all he did for me and my family. He is now retired and still going strong at 80. He gave his permission for me to thank him here publicly. THANK YOU with all my heart!!!

Presbyterian Hospital is one of the largest in New Mexico, and fully equipped with the tools of modern medicine. After I was wheeled to my room, I met my new Gastroenterologist. He shared with me that I definitely had a blockage, but considering my age, I probably had a benign tumor of the small intestines, and that any tumor in the small intestines was rarely malignant. Later that night he returned to my room with a lady surgeon---they both had long sad faces. The Gastro introduced the lady doctor and after a long pause, he broke it to me that they had found a blockage of the large colon, and that tumors in the large intestines are almost always malignant. Some people, after hearing what might be a death sentence, will stare in disbelief, some will cry, while others will get angry. In my case, I simply said with enthusiasm, "Well that explains it! What do you want to do to fix it?" I was to learn much later that they had never seen that kind of reaction and it totally threw them off-guard. When they regained their composure, they told me they wanted to operate immediately. As a side note, they also asked if I had a problem with a female surgeon. It occurred to me that a woman might be much gentler than a male doctor, and considering there weren't many female surgeons at the time, it also occurred to me that a woman in a male dominated profession would need to be exceptional just to be considered an equal. I chose to go with the lady surgeon; another vital step in the right direction. I found out later she was one of the best surgeons in the Southwest. Somehow, I knew I wasn't going to die, and I was also sure God would be watching out for me. That was proven to me so many times during that whole ordeal.

Dr. Foreman later explained to me that he had to give my previous doctor some measure of doubt, because it was rare for someone as young as I to have colon cancer. It was more common among people over 50, and that it was one of the most preventable of all cancers. Yet colon cancer was the most common cause of death from a malignancy. **That's why EVERYONE OVER 50 needs to get checked!!!!** I can personally attest to the fact that going through a colonoscopy cancer screening far out-weighs the years of recovery---if there is a recovery.

They say God has a sense of humor. I had heard the previous family doctor wanted to boost his income, so he signed up to serve in the Air Force Reserves. It was peacetime so he probably saw this as simply a weekend a month plus two weeks out of the year at the local Air Force base hospital for the duty. Shortly after he was sworn in, Iraq invaded Kuwait and he was recalled to Active Duty. He was forced to mothball his medical practice, lay off his staff, and transfer all his patients elsewhere. As he was preparing to serve on active duty and was actually traveling to his assignment, he received notice that the war was shorter than anyone expected, and he could go back to his old life. I'm sure that doctor faced a long period starting over to rebuild his medical practice.

Like my previous doctor, life would never be the same for my family and me. So much of what happened after that trip to the emergency room is somewhat clouded, but I clearly remember the vital positive steps that took me from death's door. I also had time in the hospital and while recovering at home to reflect back on what got me to that life-threatening moment. Where did this road to terminal cancer begin and more importantly, how was I going to reach my heavenly destination at an old age as God promised?

Do you know that God has given everyone the promise of living 120 years or longer? That in Old Testament times, there were people pushing 1000 years old.

So why do so many pass on before they reach 80? I'll give you a hint, the secret is in the Bible.

Part 2
Death's Road

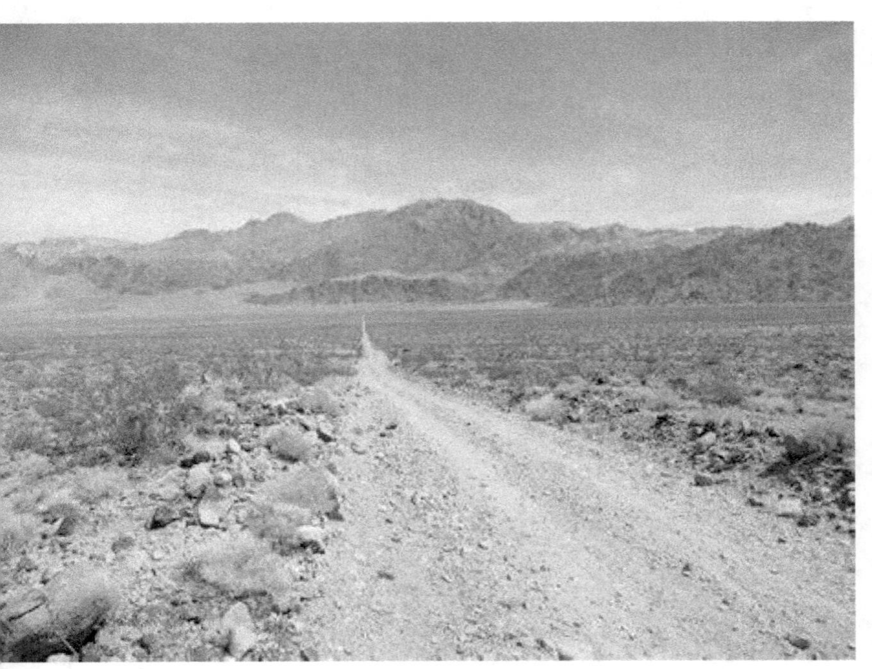

Part 2
Death's Road

Heredity

No one can choose their parents. But it's our family history that makes us who we are. In the beginning of my history, I came from an Arkansas country background. My mother was married at 15 and divorced at 18. In the middle of that short time, she became a mother of two. I am the oldest and my sister Susan is almost three years younger. Like so many poor rural families, we never saw doctors except in dire circumstances, and even then, it was often too late. It was very common back then for relatives to die of "unknown" or "natural" causes. For my sister and I, that meant we did not have any family medical history.

I was three when my natural father moved away. My sister was born months later. I didn't know anything about my father's family medical history, and my mother's side of the family didn't have a medical history, at least not for the men. The women on both sides seemed to live fairly long---well into their 80's. Their causes of death were always labeled "old age". I didn't know about the men because they had all died in their early years of "unknown" causes. My natural father lived into his early 70's and had few ailments that I was aware of, but then, he and I only had 4 or 5 occasions to talk, and that was later in my life.

A few short years after I was diagnosed with colon cancer, my natural father died from stage 4 colon cancer. He died with multiple tumors a very short time after he was diagnosed. His comment to me was that he had made medical history; he had a genetic disease that he inherited from his offspring. How much different it might have been for both of us had we known his side of the family was carrying the colon cancer gene. Apparently having the gene is only one of the contributing factors to actually having colon cancer (as is the case with many other types of cancers).

I learned later that colon cancer is one of the slowest progressing of all the cancers (there's well over 100 different types of cancer). It can also be detected early and is totally preventable. It can take 15 years for colon cancer to run its course. The insidious nature of colon cancer is that (in the absence of early diagnosis and treatment) as you are slowly dying, your body adapts, and you don't even know you have the disease until you are terminal. That is why it is so important to keep a family medical history. Both of my children started getting colonoscopies in their early 20's---the age I was diagnosed (38) minus 15 years.

To expand upon what I mentioned in Part One, I'm not a doctor, but in my research on colon cancer, I found that it is typically a disease of the elderly. It is also one of the most common forms of cancer, with the chances of someone getting it escalating after the age of 50. Did I mention **That's why <u>EVERYONE OVER 50 needs to get checked!!!!</u>**

I had the classic colon cancer symptoms, but, again, my original doctor probably ruled it out because I was only 38. That and my hard-headed attitude about seeing doctors (another family trait I inherited) were contributors to my condition becoming critical. I am amazed to hear people in the higher risk categories refusing to get colonoscopies because "it might make them feel uncomfortable".   I was awake during my first colonoscopies with only the benefit of a muscle relaxer, so I can attest that the procedure can be "uncomfortable".   The one-day preparation before the day of the procedure isn't a lot of fun either. But also from my personal experience, even after getting two colonoscopies the first year before and after surgery, one a year for the next five years, and every three years afterwards, that the checks are nothing compared to a painful and certain death! And frankly, the stuff they make you drink the night before to clean you out is worse than the colonoscopy.

Now that we know that it is in our family, so long as my children and I continue to get our routine exams, we will never get colon cancer. At least that is the assurance my Gastroenterologist gives me. Because I survived, and I get routine follow-ups, my risk of getting colon cancer again is now zero. But all of you who have never been checked are actually at a higher risk than I am. If you are over 50, you should get checked (sooner if you have a family history of cancer).

Your chances of having advanced colon cancer below the age of 50 are slim, but if you have any signs of the disease, and especially if it's in your family history, it can be detected and treated early. You don't need to turn into a hypochondriac and envision every ache and pain as cancer, but it is important that you tune in to changes in your health. Again, if it's in your family---get checked early. The rule of thumb is to take the earliest age anyone in your family was diagnosed and go back ten years beforehand to know when you should get checked. I can't speak for other forms of cancer, but if it's in your family, get checked!

Heredity is but one of the three potholes along the journey down Death's Road. The next one is diet.

****

Diet

Boy did I love to eat! I knew when I moved to the farm when I was 15 years old, that it was a physically grueling lifestyle. However, I had no idea that it was so downright brutal! The flip side of the long hours of chores was the great meals from all the home-grown food we raised. My Aunt Sylvia was famous for her cooking. When she and my Uncle Frank first bought the farm, she worked in a local diner as their cook. Eating big meals was a major part of my raising. Fresh biscuits, gravy, bacon, and eggs for breakfast; fried chicken, green beans (with bacon), peas, potatoes, corn-on-the-cob (coated with bacon grease or home-churned butter), and a half-dozen or so other items. Then after the main dishes, the meal was topped off with apple, peach, or blackberry pie for lunch; for supper (that's what we called dinner) we had the big meal of the day!

That was a diet low in fiber, rich in protein, loaded with carbohydrates---and heavy with saturated fat. If I could, I would eat ice cream

23

every single day, all day long---or more often! Matter of fact, if I was granted two wishes, the first would be to have ice cream every day for the rest of my life, and the second wish would be for "more ice cream". Even after I left the farm, I stuck with the same foods I had come to enjoy. I had no idea that a high fat, high sugar, low fiber diet like mine was deadly. How could something that tasted soooooo good be that bad? That diet is unhealthy for a number of ailments besides colon cancer. It was very common to hear of a farming community neighbor dying of a sudden stroke, heart attack, or getting diabetes. In fact, my Aunt Sylvia, who lived into her 80's, had been taking insulin for the last twenty of those years.

After I met Geneva, I found out that her mother was also a great cook. What I didn't know was that they weren't raised on the huge meals that I was used to. Geneva had grown up with her Mom, Dad, five older sisters and a brother, so they learned to eat on smaller portions. The first time I was invited to a family dinner at her house, it never occurred to me that I had eaten as much as all the others sitting at the table combined! It was a saying in my family, "get all you want, but eat all you get!" It was just considered impolite not to honor a good cook by not eating a lot of their cooking.

Geneva is now a really good cook, but that wasn't always the case. She had four older sisters who helped her Mom with all the cooking, while Geneva got to clean up afterwards (Geneva's an immaculate housekeeper). When we were dating, she invited me over twice for dinner at her apartment. One time was for enchiladas (a traditional South Texas Mexican dish that tasted amazing), and a delicious shrimp dish the second time. After we were married, she made enchiladas the first night in our new home, the shrimp dish the second night, then enchiladas, followed by shrimp, followed by... well you get the picture. That's when I found out she had limited culinary experience, so we ate out a lot!!! And the restaurant meals? Pretty much like the same ones I grew up on. I especially liked the "all-you-can-eat" buffets. (I believe I might have put some of them out of business!)

After our experience with my medical issues, we both became very good at eating healthy. Another important habit is regular fasting. In Biblical times, the Israelites would fast one or two times every single week. They would use those times to pray. I have added the practice of fasting and praying---I go an entire day (usually Mondays) without eating and only drinking water, coffee, and green tea. Then I pray---I give God thanks for all of His many blessings, especially the fact that I am able to fast voluntarily, rather than because of a food shortage. Towards the end of the day, I also pray that I make it until breakfast Tuesday morning!

I learned from doing some research (there's a ton of great books out there written by highly knowledgeable doctors) that even on a low-fat diet, your liver can become overloaded and actually stop processing fat. So instead of using fat, your body leaves it stored (ever wonder why overweight people seem to have a hard time losing the weight?). By fasting, you give your liver a chance to catch its breath and also shrink your stomach, so you'll feel fuller with smaller meals. An interesting bit of information is that the heart healthy diet is also a cancer prevention diet. A diet for prevention of colon cancer, like the healthy heart diet, also includes lots of high fiber fruits, grains, and vegetables, and very little meat or fatty foods. Another bit of interesting information---on most heart healthy/cancer prevention diets you can eat all the lettuce you want! I sure miss regular servings of ice cream.

On a serious note, death's road doesn't start at the ice cream store or dinner table. It is your lifestyle that puts a sinkhole in your path. So how did my lifestyle contribute to my bout with colon cancer? That's the last nail in the coffin I'll explain.

****

Lifestyle

Where heredity and diet combine to allow cancer to grow, the third element is lifestyle, but the trigger is stress. I read somewhere that over a billion cancer cells can fit on the head of a pin (does anyone now-a-days even know what a pin head looks like?? Just let us say they are pretty small). I also found that everyone has cancer cells in their bodies, but when you are in good physical condition, your body will kill them off (yes that means exercise). It's when you are eating poorly, not exercising, and have cancer in your genes, that your body stops fighting off the otherwise weak cancer cells. You now have all the ingredients for cancer to survive the body's defenses, grow, and become deadly. Prolonged periods of stress is a reason the body loses its ability to fight off cancer.

If we look back over my story, all the critical elements were there. I had a very bad diet and I didn't find out I had colon cancer in my family until after my second surgery (to reverse a colostomy). Both of those conditions might not have been enough to cause me to get cancer because otherwise I was healthy as a horse; the military made sure I was in good physical condition. But the stress levels started to climb as my responsibilities at work and home increased. Bad bosses, an uncertain future, financial burdens, and just life in general all added to the stress levels.

Since I have been declared cancer free (its been over 30 years), I have had prolonged periods of stress and sometimes my diet and exercise efforts have been less than they should be, but my tests continue to be good. So what's the difference since I still have the genes to get colon cancer? A couple of reasons are: one, I've drastically changed my diet; and two, I get regular checkups to make sure that any sign of cancer can be arrested before it becomes acute. But the main reason is that I have learned that when I am under stress, I just give it up to God to handle. I may still have the issues to deal with, but I don't worry about them because I have a very big God handling the stress for me so I don't have to.

Faith in God's power to heal is all important. I saved this subject last, but it is the most important part of the story to tell of my "Road" to recovery. That road wasn't an easy one for me or for my family, but there were some very crucial actions I took that saved my life. I believe that they are too important not to share. I am not qualified to give medical advice, but I know what I went through and what I did to come out of it, and I'm alive today to tell that story.

As Paul Harvey, a famous daily radio commentator, would say, "and here's the rest of the story."

Part 3
The Deadly Storm

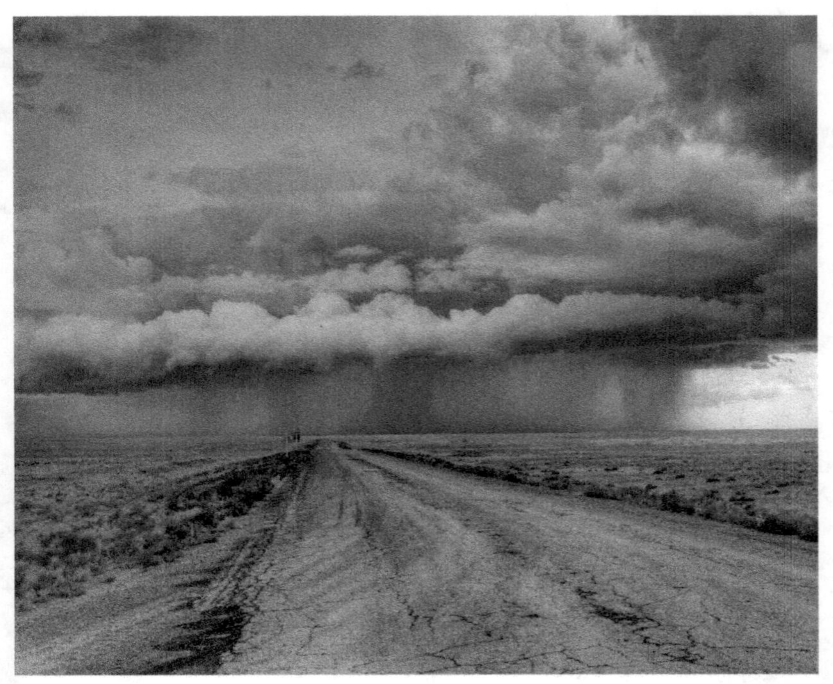

Part 3
The Deadly Storm

Within minutes of arriving at the Albuquerque Presbyterian Hospital, I found myself moved from the Emergency Room to a hospital semi-private room. After my referred Gastroenterologist came in to talk with me and Geneva, and explained that I probably had a small bowel blockage and that these types of tumors were rarely if ever cancerous; and since I was only 38 and there was no (known) family history of colon cancer, it was highly unlikely I had a problem to be too concerned about. He ordered a barium enema and xrays. That didn't sound so bad---at first, but for the uninformed like me, there can be some unexpected surprises (I'll leave it at that).

It was after 8:00 PM when the doctors broke the news to me. They explained to me that they should remove the tumor as soon as possible, and equip me with a colostomy (a colostomy is an opening in your lower abdomen that creates a bypass for your colon.) The idea of surgery didn't really bother me if it meant fixing the problem, but I wasn't too keen on a colostomy after it was explained what it was. The surgeon assured me that it would only be temporary for a short time to give the colon time to rest and heal, then she would put me all back together. So the surgery was scheduled for the next available spot on the calendar.

****

    I don't remember a lot after coming out of the surgery. I was in pretty bad shape before the surgery, so the trauma of the surgery was probably worse than it might have been. I remember the hospital room had two beds separated by a curtain. My bed was next to the window. The other patient that had been in the room before my surgery had been an older gentleman and very considerate. After the surgery was a totally different story. They had brought in a teenager who had wrecked his truck. He was banged up but would survive---his girlfriend died in the accident. Throughout the time he was in the room, there was a steady stream of high school friends, so there wasn't a lot of rest. I also got a serious infection in the surgery wound after I went home---partly from not being able to have the normal prep before the surgery, and more likely from all the germs brought in from all those high school kids.

    The comment the kid next to me made several times to his friends was, "I can't believe it, I wrecked my truck and lost my girlfriend." The emphasis was on the loss of his truck, so it appeared the truck was the greater loss to him. I can't image anything worse than losing someone you truly love. I would soon realize how much I meant to my family.

****

I could not believe all the unimaginable things hospitals can do to you. I was hooked up to a monitor that kept track of my heart rate and blood pressure; and I really believe it also tracked when you went to sleep so it could instantly alarm and wake you up. They have a tube for everything! I had a tube in my arm from the IV drip; I had a tube up my nose and into my stomach (the NG tube---don't know what that stood for, but to me it meant NOT GOOD!); and there was a tube taped to my nose for oxygen. "But thank goodness", I told myself, "they didn't stick tubes everywhere else!" After a couple of days, I found out they had even more creative things to use tubes for! Then came "everywhere else"---the bladder tube.

One evening late, after I had finally dozed off, a nurse comes in with a cart filled with various unusual devices. "Oh Lord", I said to myself, "where could they possibly stick another tube!" I didn't want to think about where the next one might go---I was running out of places. I asked her what brought her in to see me, and she told me she was there the take my vitals. "You're going to take my what?" I asked nervously. "Your vitals", was her reply. "Are you going to give them back???" I asked, now a little more than worried. She explained she was recording my vital signs and assured me it wouldn't hurt---but then so long as the morphine held out, nothing did.

I was poked, prodded, stuck, and had my vitals taken for two solid weeks. But in-between the constant visits by the nurses, I was visited by family, friends, and three wonderful preachers who prayed over me and with me. One was the Pastor of my church, another the hospital Chaplin, and the third a Charismatic preacher I had become friends with a couple of years earlier. The latter believed in the "laying on of hands" so God's healing power would flow through one who was afflicted. I'll give all three credit for getting me through that critical time in my life, but I do know now that God was the real physician in my case and that He has the power to heal---I'm living proof!

****

I really didn't want to risk another bout with colon cancer later, so I elected to go on chemotherapy as soon as I was able. The lady surgeon told me that considering my condition, she didn't think chemo was a good idea. I believe her exact words were something like, "why put yourself through unnecessary discomfort when it probably won't help." What I didn't know is the other half of the conversation she had in private with Geneva. She told her the reason she didn't think Chemo was a good idea was because she didn't expect me to make it out of the hospital alive.

When I did make it home alive and had my first follow-up, I came in with the wound issue. The medical term was "infiltrated", which means basically the tissue around the surgery site was dying. I was severely scolded for not coming in right away, and she did an impromptu surgery in her clinic right then and there! She also told me that ordinarily she would resection (put back together) the colon about six weeks after the initial surgery, but because I elected to go on Chemo, I would need to wait until after I had finished all of the treatments. That would be a year later!

****

The next sign that God was with me was the Chemo itself. The Oncologist---also a lady doctor---told me that there was still a lot of research needed to find the most effective colon cancer treatments and that I would be a good candidate for a protocol research study. Not really thinking about the implications of untried protocols, I agreed to the study (mainly because the study covered the costs of the very expensive Chemo and we were still financially strapped). The study involved three groups of test subjects. One group received a pill used to worm sheep, one had a cocktail of a Chemo enhancement drug called Leucovorin mixed with a cancer drug called fluorouracil, and the third got a placebo. My protocol was the cocktail, which turned out to be the one most effective. The pill was partially effective, but the placebo would have been no better than taking IVs of salt water.

There were other wonderful things that happened along the road to recovery. Through Geneva's employment with the government, we had a really good medical insurance plan that covered all of the medical bills. However, because I hadn't been in my new job very long working for the government, I didn't have any accrued leave—sick or vacation. That meant I would not get a paycheck for the two-week hospital stay or the six weeks of convalescence. Add another two weeks after resuming work to get the next paycheck. Around that same timeframe, the government had just started a new program where federal employees with excess annual leave could donate some of their unused hours to someone needing leave for unforeseen events like mine. Along comes Andy from my new office. Andy was an unmarried career engineer/scientist who would rather be in his lab than anywhere else. He occasionally made an appearance out of his lab, but not for long, and he never took a vacation---ever. He had maxed out the number of hours he could carry from one year to the next, so he donated several months of leave to me. What an unexpected blessing! And there were many more blessings that followed---all that I would consider gifts from God.

****

After 48 Chemo treatments consuming two hours at a time with an IV stuck in my arm, for a year (counting one-week hiatus' after each 6 weekly treatments), I was finally scheduled for my colon resection and freedom from a colostomy bag!! I hated dealing with the colostomy, but if I had been forced to have a permanent colostomy to stay alive, I would have accepted it.

There was another major miracle to come that showed again how much God will do if you put your trust in Him. It started with a prayer.

Part 4
The Prayer

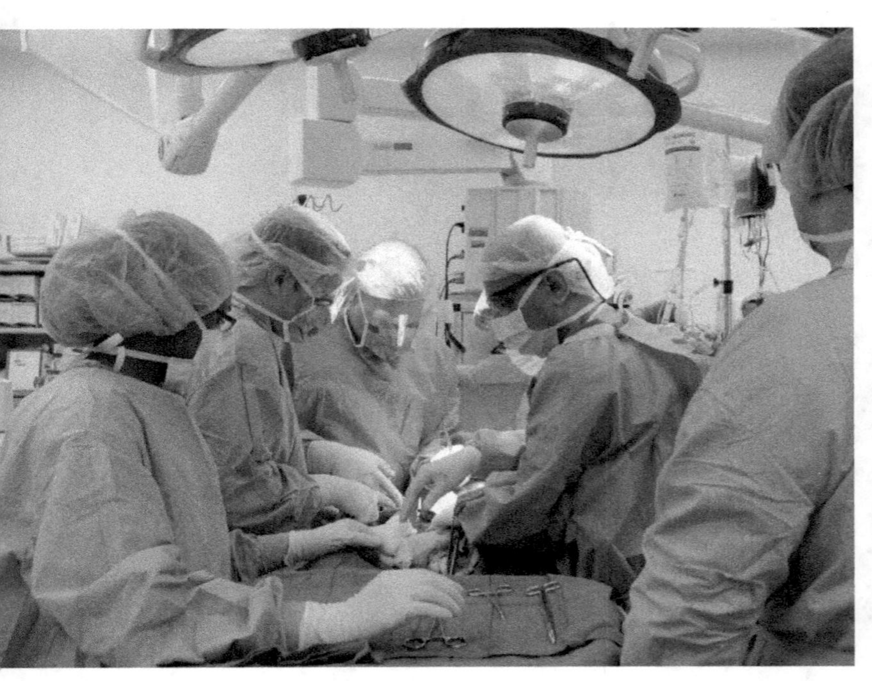

The road to recovery was a slow one that started during the original two-week hospital stay. I found out that Geneva had convened a prayer meeting on my behalf, so while I had preachers with me asking God to heal me, and while I was praying and believing I would be healed, a group of friends were also praying for me. Prayer does work!

During the six-week convalescing at home, I had time to read, rest, and to exercise. One of the books I read was the book, "Love, Medicine, and Miracles", by Dr. Bernie Siegel. Dr. Siegel was a surgeon that discovered that some patients who he believed would survive a life-threatening condition would not, while others who he had written off would survive and do well afterwards (like myself). He found out that the one single factor that was common in those two groups of patients was their expectations. Those who believed they would die, did; those who believed they would live, survived. In my world, that translates to Faith. I believed 100% that God would heal me---and He did!

One of the interesting things that I read in Dr. Siegel's book was that when you are under anesthesia, you are subject to hypnotic

suggestion. Apparently, the subconscious never sleeps and remembers what is said during a surgery even if the patient does not recollect anything. So it occurred to me, that having a healing prayer said over me while I was under, would open up yet another channel to God. Before my second surgery, I wrote a prayer that began:
"I will heal quickly with minimum discomfort." I included a line about living a long, productive, and successful life. Another that mentioned getting back into a solid weight training program. Since I had been an amateur bodybuilder trying to get bigger muscles, I even included something about becoming bigger than I had ever thought possible. I had no idea how powerful that simple prayer would be.

When it came time for the second surgery, I asked the doctor to read the prayer I had written, and she said she would. Now understand, when you go under, they can do or say anything, and you wouldn't really know for sure if they followed your instructions. When I was back from recovery afterwards, the doctor told me everything went well and to make sure the prayer "stuck" she instructed the anesthesiologist not to administer the standard amnesia drug that wipes your memory of going into surgery. This was apparently the case, because I remembered everything up to counting down from 10,9,8..... For the first surgery, I remembered nothing from immediately beforehand. The surgery went so well that she had time left over, so she gave me a tummy tuck! She also said she knew I would be back to lifting weights, so to make sure I didn't rip something, she sewed me up with rope.

****

Now the miracle. The prayer they read to me started out, "I will heal quickly with minimum discomfort". The very first day out of surgery, I got out of bed with my IV stand in tow, and went for a walk. Presbyterian hospital is huge, and my floor was a perfect walking path. I could walk all along the perimeter in a big circle. As I walked, I kept track of the laps. I felt so good, I didn't stop. For the next several days, I walked---and walked---and walked! Altogether that week, I walked (as best I could calculate) thirty-three miles.

At one point, the staff couldn't find me so I was paged over the PA system to please come back to my room so they could take my vitals (they agreed not to keep them this go around). I was amused by the irony of needing to check to see if I was alive when I was obviously full of life. They also told me to PLEASE take a shower.

The surgery was on a Monday. On Wednesday, the nurse removed my bandage to find that in just two short days, the scab had flaked off and there was nothing left on my abdomen but a thin red line. The wound had totally healed! Shortly after that, all of the tubes came out and I was allowed to eat soup and jello. My appetite had roared back to life, and it was painful to walk the halls seeing trays of uneaten solid foods on the floor outside of the rooms. By the end of the week, they kicked me out---I was making all the other patients feel bad with me walking around.

The walking didn't end when I came home. I lived near the mountain trails, so I was doing a two-mile hike almost every day. In a very short time, I was back at work and feeling better than I had in years. It was 1988 when I was first hospitalized for "terminal" colon cancer. I have been cancer free from the day after that first surgery. I also adapted the prayer I had written, and began a habit of reading it every morning when I first got up and every evening before going to bed. As my life changed over the years, I have adapted the twice daily prayer and continue to read it.

Now, your task is to write a personal prayer affirming your total healing. If you are healthy, there wouldn't be any harm in writing your own daily prayer that means something to you. It should be personal and meaningful. You may want to write two versions. If you are having surgery and will be under anesthesia, you would style the prayer for whoever is saying the prayer over you. For example, the prayer I asked to have

read over me for my colostomy reversal started out:
"<u>You</u> will recover quickly with minimal discomfort."

Write the other version that you read twice daily to yourself in the first person using such words as "**I AM**", and "**I Will**". The first line should declare your healing, such as:
"**I AM** totally healed of cancer and **I WILL** live a long, healthy, and happy life."

In the Bible Book of Exodus, we learn the two most powerful words in the entire universe are: "**I AM**".

Exodus 3:13-14

13 Moses said to God, "Suppose I go to the Israelites and say to them, 'The God of your fathers has sent me to you,' and they ask me, 'What is his name?' Then what shall I tell them?"

14 God said to Moses, "**I AM WHO I AM**. This is what you are to say to the Israelites: '**I AM** has sent me to you.'"

When you speak the words, "**I AM** totally healed of cancer, you are affirming that you are now healed. When you say these words in prayer, not only are you affirming your belief that you are, in fact, healed, you are invoking the infinite power of

God (the **Great I AM**) and that power will come over you.

Your twice daily prayer should also contain petitions for aspects of your life you want to change or improve upon. These might appear to be selfish, but Jesus, Himself, said in James 4:2: "You do not have because you do not ask God."

I not only asked for healing, I asked to become bigger and stronger than I ever believed possible. At the time, this sounded pretty reasonable since I was still wanting to improve as a weightlifter. This is one thing I should have thought through a little further! The part about becoming stronger was a good thing, but when I ballooned to 265 pounds and was on track to hit 300, I had to modify it to say I would be a lean and muscled 225 pounds. So, a word of caution, be careful what you ask for, because our God is a very giving God, and he will give you what you ask. But more importantly, never forget to thank Him for granting you a longer and blessed life.

Some of the Things I Remember
(Geneva's Testimony)
By
Geneva E. Boyd

While James (I don't call him Hoss!!) was working in Ft Worth he would write me letters telling how tired he was and that he didn't have any energy. I also remember the struggles we were going through. We couldn't join him in Ft Worth because our home hadn't sold. We were just praying for God to give James a job or to have our home sell (even though it would be at a loss) so we could get united as a family again. James finally got a job back in Albuquerque at the Air Force Weapons Lab and we were all rejoicing. We were so excited. That Christmas, our son James and daughter Missy helped me decorate and put up all the luminarias on top of the roof. It was bitter cold that night but we did it so we could have everything beautiful when James drove home.

Looking back, I realize God had a reason for us not selling our home at that time. With James getting a steady paycheck, we could stay in the home we had built. When it did come time to move, it was for a promotion back to my home state of Texas, and our home sold at the very peak of the market---a window that was only open for a few short months. I did not realize James was actually dying when he came home. I now see where God made it possible for James to get the best professional healthcare he needed at the time with little or no cost to us because of the HMO and the wonderful co-workers we had (especially the one who donated so much leave to him.) Praise God!!!

Fast forward to next year:
James had been even more tired as the weeks went by. Our family doctor at the time told us James had an ulcer. We agreed with the diagnosis and believed that was true with all the stress we had been through. We had been planning to visit James' family in Oklahoma for Thanksgiving that year and drove up to see them. We made the drive and were sleeping in his brother's travel trailer parked next to their house. We had eaten Thanksgiving dinner and finally had gone to bed so we could get up early to leave and come back home the next day. That night James started feeling sick and threw up all night. We thought it might be food poisoning even though none of us had gotten sick. We drove our 10 hours home but he was still tired and weak. But he later faithfully went to work and all through December continued to get weaker and lost weight. We were getting ready to change health plans to an HMO starting in January. As it turned out, James still wasn't feeling great but didn't want to go see our former

doctor since the old doctor was not on the new plan. Despite not feeling good or looking good he still managed to find strength to go to work but would come home, barely eat, and just lay on the couch. That was not at all normal for James---he never did that! My sister and her husband came up from Texas to visit us for Christmas that year. James hardly ate anything for Christmas dinner, and I remember my sister and I were talking, trying to figure out what might be wrong with him. We were concerned he might have stomach cancer. He was losing a lot of weight and his skin color was gray---he just wasn't his friendly jovial self.

Happy New Year! Finally, January was here, and we had a new Health Plan (an HMO). What a blessing because it covered 100% of our medical expenses. I looked up new doctors and found Dr. Robert Foreman. James was still hesitant to go to the doctor but did. Dr. Foreman was on vacation, so James ended up seeing his Physician's Assistant (PA). James told him about the ulcer diagnosis and when the PA asked if the ulcer had healed, James told him no. The PA prescribed medicine and told us if James wasn't feeling better in 10 days to come back.

After a couple of days, James was actually feeling better. I was thrilled and relieved. Knowing how much he loved to eat, I fixed him a huge meal that night. I believe it was steak, baked potato and salad and I even fixed him a milkshake. It seemed he was back to normal. He ate well and I was thankful that things might be improving. That was until he woke me up in the middle of the night throwing up black matter. He was also in a lot of abdominal pain. I wanted to take him to the emergency room but (being stubborn), he wanted to wait and call Dr. Foreman in the morning. I went to work and told my supervisor that I was calling the Dr. and needed to take my husband in---I believed James was dying. I called Dr. Foreman's office and told them James' symptoms and they were able to see him immediately. When I got home to pick him up, James was so pale and weak. He had no color.

Dr. Foreman had not seen James prior to then, but by that time, James' stomach was very distended (swollen)---he looked like he was 9 months pregnant. Dr. Foreman immediately told us he was calling the hospital to admit James and to run a series of tests. So we went directly from Dr. Foreman's office to Albuquerque's Presbyterian Hospital.

Soon after we arrived, they gave James a barium enema for the x-rays, but the technician told me they were unable to complete the test because James had a blockage. An excellent surgeon was contacted by Dr. Foreman, who met with us at the hospital. She told us that, due to the blockage, she needed to operate. James' response was a simple, "Well, Let's get it done." He was so upbeat and happy because they finally figured out what was going on with him! I'm sure that wasn't the reaction the doctor expected.

The day of the surgery, several of my co-workers showed up to give us support. We prayed together for James to come through, and the surgery was successful. However, the surgeon told me later in private that James' colon had ruptured, and he had peritonitis---a severe infection of the colon lining. It was the worst the doctor had ever seen and that I should call the family together, go home, and get all of our things in order because James only had about 2 weeks to live.

I'm not sure she ever told James that, but I was devastated. I didn't want him or our children to know. I was trying to stay positive and faithful especially when I was with James at the hospital. The whole time, I was praying and trusting God. The doctor told James the next day that he had stage 4 colon cancer and that there was no need for chemotherapy since James wouldn't live long enough for the chemo to do any good. Even though she was a superb surgeon, she did not have the best of bed-side manners. James was not a cooperative patient and insisted on seeing an oncologist just the same---he was not going to give up that easily. Thank God he didn't give up and insisted on seeing the oncologist!

In walks another great doctor who was a wonderful oncologist. She told James chemotherapy would be worth it because "what do you have to lose" (and after it was apparent that after two weeks, James was improving). She put him on an experimental protocol cancer drug and it is true, "with God all things are possible". James is here today because of God's healing powers, the HMO, the Doctors provided to us, our family, our prayers, and our faith.

I also remember how sad our children were during that time. Our son, James, was very athletic and involved in school activities and baseball. I was going through his notebooks a few years later and discovered a note he had written to God asking him to help his dad get better because he didn't know what he would do if something happened to his dad---he would have had some pretty big shoes to fill. I didn't realize what an impact this had on all of us until I read that. Our daughter, Missy, was also going through a lot of difficulties and stress as a young teenager during that time. I realized that God brought James (Senior) through all that for a reason and it's because we all needed him. He was our strength and the backbone of our family, and we relied heavily on him.

Again, looking back I now see God's plan in our lives. His was a good plan and for a special purpose. We have so much to be grateful for and especially praise God for always being there and loving us so much.

Epilogue

The story of Hezekiah in the Old Testament Book of 2nd Kings is of a good king who is told he will soon die. Just as what I experienced, Hezekiah believed God could change His mind, so he prayed to live longer. Because he had been a righteous king, God granted him fifteen more years. In my case, I have been granted twice that and more! Maybe it's because I still have a lot of work to do. Over the past years since that dark day in Albuquerque, I have published many books and nationally published articles; seen my son and daughter graduate both high school and college; walked my daughter down the aisle at her wedding; and later to get to know two beautiful granddaughters; and was there for my son's wedding as well. I've served my country and retired with thirty years of Active and Reserve Air Force duty; and grown a company that as of this writing is still in business after twenty years. But probably the most special achievement is that I am still married to that special woman who stood by me during those really bad times (and a few bad times before and afterwards), and in 2024 (the year of this printing), we celebrate our Fiftieth Wedding Anniversary--- another major miracle!!!

Our God is a great and giving God. He has the power to heal if you will but only believe and receive His gifts.

Special (Restricted) Reproduction Permission

Any religious non-profit organization may request permission to locally reproduce this publication in any form under the understanding that said reproduction is for the sole purpose of sharing this work with those and their families going through a life-threatening event, and not for a commercial purpose. Permission (if requested) may also be granted to allow the non-profit to accept gifts for this publication to benefit the lives of those who they serve.

Please include a short description of what form the reproduction will be made (electronic or print; excerpts or complete publication), how the publication will be used, those it will be shared with, and any information you might believe to be pertinent.

Address your requests to:
Your House in Order
c/o James A. Hoss Boyd, LtCol, USAF (Retired)
PO Box 312287
New Braunfels, Texas 78131-2287

About the Author
James A. "Hoss" Boyd, Lt. Col, USAF. (Retired)

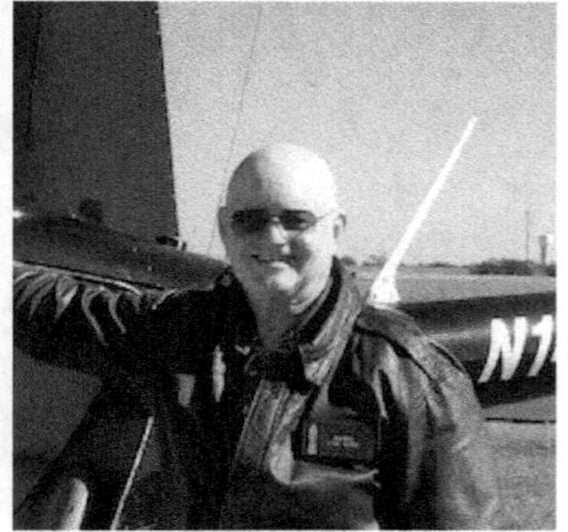

Although Hoss has a number of achievements to his credit, the most significant is surviving a near-fatal bout with colon cancer. Equally significant is him being able to live to celebrate three (or more) decades of marriage to his wife, Geneva; see his children marry wonderful spouses and go out into the world to have families of their own; then see his daughter and son grow and achieve at levels even higher than Hoss'.

Hoss continues to share his story with those battling cancer.

Life is something that can neither be bought nor sold; it can only be shared with others. Author Unknown